Table of Contents

Introduction

A fruitarian diet, also called a fructarian diet, is a form of vegan diet that is generally limited to eating fruits. The definition of what is a fruit often varies among fruitarians also called fructarians or frugivores. Some adhere to a strict interpretation, consuming only fruits from plants and trees. Some fruitarians include berries in their diet, others broaden the definition to include nuts and seeds, while yet others include some food that is commonly thought of as vegetables, including peppers, tomatoes, cucumbers, and avocados.

What is fruitarian diet

The fruitarian diet is a subset of the vegan diet and it works just the way it sounds—you eat mostly (or all) fruit on the fruitarian diet. The fruitarian diet is one of the most restrictive eating patterns out there, and the risk of malnourishment is high, despite the nutritional quality of most fruits.

A fruitarian diet means that raw fruit should make up 50–75% of your foods consumed. The strictest fruitarians, however, may eat up to 90% fruit. The fruitarian diet is nothing new, although its popularity has soared in recent years along with vegan diets and raw food diets.

Following a vegan diet means eating only plant-based foods. A raw food diet is essentially a vegan diet (though some may consume raw eggs and dairy) that excludes foods that have been heated, refined, pasteurized, or otherwise treated. Fruitarianism means eating only raw fruit, nuts, and seeds.

Types

There are different types of fruit diet, and some are more restrictive than others.Some people on a fruitarian diet only eat what drops from the tree or plant, to avoid picking or harvesting. The goal is to refrain from doing anything that would harm the plant.

Other people avoid grains, nuts, and seeds because of beliefs about what is natural for a human to eat.

Some fruitarians eat only raw fruit before a certain time, such as noon or a point in the evening, after which they will introduce other foods.

Others take a more flexible approach and may eat small amounts of the following throughout the day:

- nuts
- seeds
- pulses
- grains
- vegetables

Overall, fruit-based diets are extremely restrictive and do not provide key nutrients. Also, for some people, following very restrictive diets contributes to an unhealthy relationship with food.

A person can often benefit from following a less restrictive diet that still includes plenty of fruits and vegetables and few, if any, processed foods.

Health Benefits

1. Encourages Whole, Nutritious Foods

Fruits are well-known for their healthful properties, including high antioxidant content and high concentration of vitamins, minerals, electrolytes, phytonutrients, and fiber. The high fiber content of fruit also promotes satiety, which could lead to weight loss.

2. Promotes Hydration

In addition to their high nutrient density, fruits also contain a lot of water. Eating such large quantities of fruit can aid in hydration.

Fruitarianism encourages people to eat when they are hungry and stop when they are full. In other words, fruitarians eat intuitively. When eaten in moderation, fruit can be a very healthy part of a nutritious diet. Some benefits from eating fruit include:

Fruits contain fiber, which can help lower your cholesterol and encourage regular bowel movements. Apples, pears, blackberries, and raspberries are examples of fruits high in dietary fiber.

Oranges, red peppers, and strawberries are examples of fruits that contain lots of vitamin C. This helps keep teeth and gums healthy. Vitamin C also supports the immune system.

Bananas, guavas, cantaloupe, and mangos are examples of fruits higher in potassium. Potassium can help maintain a healthy blood pressure and regulate fluid balance in the body.

Oranges and tropical fruits such as mangos are high in folate. This can help the body produce red blood cells. Folate also supports healthy fetal development. Looking for fruits that are low in sugar? Try these.

Black plums, prunes, and all berries are examples of fruits rich in antioxidants. Antioxidants limit the production of free radicals. They can protect your skin and fight off illness.

Benefits

The benefits of a fruitarian diet are mostly promoted by people on the diet, rather than scientific research. These benefits include increased mental power and clarity, creativity, happiness, energy, confidence, self-esteem, and concentration. Physical health benefits, according to the Fruitarian Foundation, include preventing and curing cancer, constipation, insomnia, depression, and digestive problems, weight loss, wound healing, strengthening the immune system, reducing or eliminating menstruation, increasing sexual vitality, improvements in the health and appearance of skin, hair, eyes, and nails, improving muscle coordination, and the ability to control addictions to alcohol, drugs, and tobacco. The United States Department of Agriculture recommends fruit be included in daily meal planning, although the amount depends on age, gender, weight, height, level of physical activity, and weight loss goals. It must be noted that there is no scientific evidence that eating a fruit-only diet can cure any disease.

1. Fruit is the best tasting raw food and eating fruit is a pleasant experience.
2. It helps cleanse the body of toxins.
3. Fruit grown and sold locally is environmentally friendly.
4. It promotes weight loss
5. It can improve the function of the respiratory system.
6. It sharpens the senses, especially those of taste and smell.
7. It reduces the amount of water a person needs to drink since most fruit has a high water content

What are the potential risks?

Several nutrients that are vital for overall health are lacking in a fruit-based diet.

This includes:

- protein
- fat
- calcium

- B vitamins
- omega-3 fatty acids

Due to the diet's highly restrictive nature, malnourishment is a significant concern. Your body might even go into starvation mode. This means that your metabolism will slow as it attempts to hold onto your nutritional stores and conserve energy. You may also experience anemia, fatigue, and a reduced immune system. Over time, the lack of calcium can lead to osteoporosis.

A fruit-based diet is also very heavy on sugar, even though it's a natural source. This may make it a poor choice for people with diabetes, prediabetes, polycystic ovarian syndrome, or insulin resistance.

There aren't any ironclad rules to follow, so you may be able to adapt the fruit diet to your specific nutritional needs. Limiting your fruit intake to 50 percent and adding protein sources, such as nuts or vegetarian-approved supplements, may help balance out the nutritional deficits inherent in the fruit diet.

Function

There are as many reasons for being a fruitarian as there are variations of the fruitarian diet. One reason is the opposition to killing animals for food, another is opposition to consuming any products that come from animals. Other reasons include opposition to killing any plant for food, health benefits, environmental concerns, and spiritual beliefs. The primary function of a fruitarian diet is to promote health and energy. Once someone adopts a fruit diet, they become physically, mentally, emotionally, and spiritually healthier, according to the Fruitarian Foundation (http://www.fruitarian.com). The foundation's philosophy states that fruitarians develop a fine-tuned body and experience few or no headaches, develop a greater resistance to illness, pain, and aging, and need less sleep. 'The proper application of fruitarian dietary and lifestyle is calculated to allow the human to produce healthy offspring, live more than 100 years of age, be free of all disease, and only Lsquo;mature' while not aging, as most people think of it, and die a natural death in their sleep,' according to a statement on the foundation's Website. 'Man cannot eat of everything and maintain his good health. Man was created to eat of the fruits of the trees.

What You Need to Know

Similar to the proponents of the paleo diet, many followers of the fruitarian diet tout the eating plan as the original diet of humankind. Some fruitarians are motivated by a desire to not kill any living organism, even plantsh ence, why they eat only the fruit of a plant.

There isn't any specific meal-timing for the fruitarian diet. The plan actually encourages you to eat intuitively or only eat when you're hungry and stop when you're full. There aren't any hard-and-fast rules about how much or when to eat on the fruitarian diet. In this case, it's recommended that you focus on eating at least three full meals each day, with snacks in between if you get hungry. A benefit of intuitive eating is that you're free to follow your hunger cues.

There are countless ways to modify the fruitarian diet, which may make the diet healthier. For instance, you could eat a fruit-based diet and still include other essential food groups such as whole grains and protein. A modified fruitarian diet might look like this:

- 50% fruit
- 20% plant-based protein (e.g., tempeh, soy, seitan)
- 20% vegetables
- 10% whole grains (e.g., oats, wheat, bulgur, quinoa, etc.)

Adding other foods to the fruitarian diet ensures a better nutritional composition and decreases the risk of nutrient deficiencies and health complications.

What to Eat

To be a fruitarian, at least 50–75% of your calories must come from raw fruit, such as bananas, papayas, grapes, apples, and berries. Usually, the other 25–50% of your calories would come from nuts, seeds, vegetables, and whole grains. Strict fruitarians, however, may eat up to 90% fruit and just 10% nuts and seeds.

The fruitarian diet typically revolves around these seven fruit groups:

- **Acid fruits:** citrus, cranberries, pineapples
- **Subacid fruits**: sweet cherries, raspberries, figs
- **Sweet fruits:** bananas, grapes, melons
- **Oily fruits**: avocados, coconuts, olives
- **Vegetable fruits:** peppers, tomatoes, cucumbers, squash
- **Nuts:** hazelnuts, cashews, almonds, pistachios, walnuts
- **Seeds:** sunflower, pumpkin, squash

1. Fruit

A fruitarian diet encourages a variety of fruits, including exotic ones like rambutan, mangosteen, passionfruit, jackfruit, durian, longan, and snake fruit. Of course, more common fruits such as bananas, pears, apples, oranges, and berries are also encouraged. Fruit also includes foods we don't usually think of as fruits: tomatoes, cucumbers, peppers, avocados, squashes, and olives.

2. Nuts and Seeds

Nuts and seeds are technically a part of the fruits of plants, so fruitarians are encouraged to fill in the rest of their diets with foods like pepitas, sunflower seeds, walnuts, and almonds.

3. Some Vegetables

It isn't recommended that anyone follow a 100% fruit diet. Many fruitarians consume some vegetables, mostly leafy greens.

4. Beverages

Fruitarians can drink coconut water, fresh fruit juices, and water. Coffee is permitted based on an individual's preference.

What Not to Eat

1. Animal Protein

A fruitarian does not consume any animal protein. Eggs, poultry, pork, and beef aren't options for fruitarians.

2. Dairy Products

Just like animal protein, dairy products aren't permitted for the fruitarian diet. Milk, yogurt, cheese, or any other animal dairy products are not allowed. Some fruitarians are known to drink almond, cashew, or coconut milk in place of cow's or goat's milk.

3. Grains

Grains and grain products are not allowed on the fruitarian diet, and this includes sprouted grain products.

5. Starches

You might think that potatoes would be allowed on the fruitarian diet, but that isn't the case. Fruitarians don't eat any kind of tuber or potato.

6. Beans and Legumes

A true fruitarian diet does not include any beans or legumes, including chickpeas, lentils, peas, soybeans, and peanuts.

7. Processed Foods

Processed foods are not permitted on the fruitarian diet. This means shopping only the perimeter of your grocery store or at your local farmers' market.

Research and general acceptance

There is little, if any, scientific research that supports fruitarianism as a healthy lifestyle, especially over the long-term, unless foods such as beans, green vegetables, soy, and whole grains are included in the diet. However, there is much scientific documentation on the benefits of a vegetarian diet. There is general and widespread disapproval of an all-fruit diet by the medical, scientific, fitness, and vegetarian communities. Many people experience positive results after initially going on a fruitarian diet but over time develop health problems, including emaciation, constant hunger, weakness, and fatigue.

One-day meal plan

The following is a typical one-day meal plan from the Fruitarian Foundation for a fruitarian diet:

Early morning (6-9 a.m.): The juice of three to five lemons immediately upon waking, raisins, and an unlimited amount of melon or melon juice

Midmorning (9 a.m. to 12 p.m.): An unlimited amount of apples, pineapple, figs, pears, grapes, yellow plums, lima beans, kiwi, and cucumber

Noon (12-3 p.m.): Oranges or tangerines, peaches, apricots, and papayas in any amount desired

Midafternoon (3-6 p.m.): Mango, cherries, strawberries, red plums, persimmons, pomegranates, watermelon, and tomatoes

Evening 6-9 p.m.): Grapes, blackberries, and raspberries

Late evening (9 p.m. to 12 a.m.): Mango, cherries, strawberries, red plums, persimmons, pomegranates, watermelon, and tomatoes

Items that can be eaten at anytime are bananas, coconut, organic olives, ripe avocados, any type of raw nuts, and lemon juice. The only items that should be consumed from midnight to 3 a.m., if desired, are four to six passion fruit, a small amount of water (if needed), and lemon juice.

How to transition into a fruit diet

If the diet appeals to you, proceed slowly. Rather than start all at once, make a gradual transition away from your current eating patterns.

This may mean giving up:

- alcohol
- animal products
- grains
- processed foods
- caffeine

You should also begin adding:

- raw fruits
- nuts
- seeds
- vegetables

Fruitarians typically eat freely from multiple fruit groups. You may wish to stick to a three-meal-a-day plan, or build in four to five smaller meals throughout the day.

The fruit groups to choose from include:

1. acidic fruits, such as oranges, grapefruit, tomatoes, berries, plums, and cranberries
2. sub-acidic fruits, such as apples, apricots, raspberries, and cherries
3. oily fruits, such as avocados, olives, and coconuts
4. sweet fruits, such as bananas, dates, figs, and grapes
5. starchy fruits, such as squash
6. melons of all kinds
7. vegetable-fruits, such as cucumbers and bell peppers

If you can, opt for organic fruits whenever possible. And if you want them to last longer, make sure you're storing your fruits correctly!

You should also drink water, coconut water, or 100 percent fruit juice throughout the day.

Pros and cons of fruitarian diet

Fruitarian Diet Pros:

We all know fruits have many health benefits. Here we are going to know about fruitarian diet pros. These are...

1. One of the most popular Fruitarian Diet pros is it helps to reduce weight and also helps to prevent weight gain.
2. Improving digestion is another fruitarian diet pros. Fruits are rich in micronutrient which can be digested easily.
3. Fruits are rich in fiber which reduce problems of constipation.
4. Fruits are all natural food that works as an anti-aging agent. Maintaining a fruitarian diet helps you to age slow.
5. fruitarian diet increases mental power.
6. Following the fruitarian diet also helps to boost mood and makes you happy.
7. Fruits are the best friend of our beauty. Fruitarian diet makes skin, hair eyes and nails healthy and glowy.

8. Many people said that fruit diet is helpful for preventing Cancer.
9. Fruitarian diet Improves cholesterol levels, It reduces bad cholesterol and increases good cholesterol.
10. Fruitarian diet detoxifies our body and makes us healthy.

1. Fruits are relatively cheap

One advantage of the fruitarian diet is that fruits are usually rather cheap and a diet that relies solely on fruits can save you plenty of money. However, there is a caveat to this. It vastly depends on which kind of fruit you want to eat.

There are also some exotic fruits and depending on your taste and your preferences, you can also spend lots of money on a fruit-based diet.

2. Possible increase in life expectancy

Since fruits are considered to be healthy, a fruitarian diet might also increase your life expectancy. Whether this is actually true or not is hard to say. There had been many studies trying to find answers to this question.

However, there are so many other factors that affect life expectancy that it is almost impossible to figure out the true effect of fruitarianism. For instance, fruitarian's might be more aware of their health and willing to work out more compared to non-fruitarian people. Thus, although they might have a higher life expectancy on average, this might rather be due to their higher awareness regarding their health than on the fruitarian lifestyle itself.

3. Fruitarians tend to suffer less from overweight

Compared to other diet forms, people who engage in the fruitarian diet are known to be rather slim and do not suffer from overweight or obesity too often. This may be due to the fact that fruitarians might care more about their nutrition and will therefore refrain from eating too much.

4. May have a positive effect on your health

The fruitarian diet is also often associated with a healthy lifestyle and is also known to improve peoples' health, at least if this form of diet is executed properly. The fruitarian diet can lower the risk for hearth conditions and for several forms of cancer.

However, it may also potentially harm our body since there is also a lack of vitamins and other nutrients. Therefore, in order to stay healthy, it is necessary for fruitarians to rely on food supplements to get sufficient amounts of certain nutrients.

5. May improve digestion

Fruits are also known to be quite beneficial for our digestive system. They usually improve the conditions in our gut flora. Since a working digestive system is crucial to assure our health, fruitarianism may not only be a great way to improve our digestive system, but also to improve our overall health level.

6. We could feed more people on a global scale

Compared to a conventional diet that also contains meat, the fruitarian lifestyle would also make it possible to feed more people on our planet.

Since for the production of one calory of meat, multiple calories of plants have to be used, meat consumption is quite inefficient from a calory perspective.

7. Less meat is needed

If more people switch to a fruitarian diet, also the overall demand for meat would decrease. This would be quite beneficial for many people on our planet since meat consumption implies many serious environmental problems. Also, fewer animals have to die if we refrained from eating meat and consumed fruits instead.

8. Need for factory farming decreases

In order to meet our enormous global food supply, a high fraction of our meat comes from factory farming. However, factory farming is often criticized since it implies a quite poor treatment of animals.

If more people switch from a meat-based to a fruitarian diet, the need for factory farming would decrease, which would be quite desirable from an ethical standpoint since we could save plenty of animals to grow up under those adverse conditions.

9. Fewer antibiotics have to be used

If we are able to reduce our overall meat consumption through a switch to fruitarianism, also fewer antibiotics have to be used. Antibiotics are a quite convenient way to keep a high number of animals on a confined space healthy in the factory farming process. However, this excessive use of antibiotics also implies serious issues.

For instance, our medical treatment often relies on antibiotics to cure diseases. We as humans can become antibiotic-resistant through the consumption of meat that is contaminated with high levels of antibiotics.

If this is the case, the medical treatment with antibiotics might no longer work properly and many people might die due to this issue in the long run.

Therefore, it might make sense for you to switch from a meat-based to a fruitarian diet in order to avoid antibiotic resistance.

10. Fish stocks may be able to recover

Overfishing has also been a big problem over the past decades. Many fish species are now endangered and may even be at risk to become extinct in the near future if we continue our fishing behavior like we do today. Hence, it is crucial to take measures in order to stabilize our fish stocks.

Apart from the protection of certain fish species, another effective way to reduce the overfishing problem would be to switch from a conventional to a fruitarian diet since by doing so, fewer amounts of fish would be consumed since fish is not allowed in a fruitarian diet.

FRUITARIAN DIET CONS:

Many people say that a fruitarian diet has more risks than health benefits. Now that we know which are the fruitarian diet pros we should also know now the Fruitarian Diet cons. So let's know which are those Fruitarian diet cons. See those below...

1. While there are some people think that this diet could lose weight, some people also think that fruitarian diet can lead to weight gain as fruits are rich in natural sugars and having a large portion of fruit can put on a lot of weight.
2. Fruits contain so much sugar that eating too much can negatively affect blood sugar levels. This diet can be dangerous for

diabetic patients and also increase the risk for non-diabetic people too.

3. Fruits are high in sugar content that can put you at high risk for tooth decay. Some fruits, such as oranges, are highly acidic and can erode tooth enamel.

4. People who follow fruitarians diet frequently have low levels of vitamin B12, calcium, vitamin D, iodine and omega-3 fatty acids. That leads them to various health issues.

5. Fruitarians diet have low vitamin B12 levels which lead them to anemia, tiredness, lethargy and immune system dysfunction.

6. Fruitarian diet is low calcium that can cause osteoporosis.

7. The only solid protein sources allowed on most fruitarian diets are certain nuts and seeds in small amounts. Consuming an all-fruit or almost all-fruit diet makes it very easy to fall short on daily protein needs, resulting in protein deficiency.

8. The fruitarian diet restricts your fare to just fruits. Just eating one kind of food will make you long for other types to add to your diet.

You might start dreaming and craving about that juicy cheeseburger a lot more.

1. Problems with high levels of acidity

Apart from the advantages of fruitarianism, there are also some problems related to a fruitarian diet. One downside of fruitarianism is that it might lead to problems with your stomach.

For instance, through the consumption of large amounts of fruits, the acidity levels in your stomach will be quite high. Some people are quite sensitive to high acidity levels and might suffer from serious discomfort.

Moreover, excessive acidity may also lead to a state where the body might no longer be able to process the vitamins and nutrients properly, which may lead to additional health issues in the long run.

2. Vitamin deficiencies

In general, fruitarians are at greater risk of vitamin and nutrient deficiency compared to people engaging in conventional diets. There are some components in meat that are crucial for our health that are only insufficiently available through fruits.

3. Challenge to implement in your daily life

It might also be quite a challenge to live a fruitarian lifestyle, especially in regions where it is not popular yet. For instance, if you grow up in a region where meat is quite popular and everything else is considered to be dodgy, chances are that you might have a rather hard time to effectively practice a fruitarian diet.

It may also be quite hard to find a store which supplies you with certain kinds of fruits that are needed for your diet to work. Thus, depending on your area and the level of tolerance towards fruitarianism, it may be hard for you to implement this kind of lifestyle in an efficient manner.

4. High level of confinement

Since the fruitarian lifestyle is mainly based on fruits and nuts, you will be quite confined regarding your choices in the grocery store. On the one hand, it may be hard to refrain from all the other delicious foods that would be available to you.

On the other hand, you might also have problems to find a store that offers a variety of foods that are suitable for a fruitarian lifestyle since some exotic fruits might be quite hard to get. Therefore, you might be pretty confined in your choices and may also have to take additional efforts to get everything you need for your diet.

5. Physical and mental power may suffer

Depending on your level of experience and your knowledge regarding your fruitarian diet, you might also suffer from a decline of mental as well as of physical power. If you are a beginner in the fruitarian world, chances are that your nutrition will not be well-composed and that you will suffer from a lack of certain nutrients and minerals.

This will take away some of your power since our body only works optimally if it gets an optimal nutrient mix. Therefore, especially if people are inexperienced with the fruitarian lifestyle, they might suffer from a serious drop in power.

6. Motivation may be a problem

It may also be quite hard to stay on track with your fruitarian diet. Especially if you love meat and consumed plenty of it in the past, it will be hard for you to refrain from buying it in the long run.

Chances are that one day, you may break with the rules of fruitarianism and get yourself a nice steak. Thus, it will also need a great level of motivation to refrain from meat and other delicious foods in the long run.

7. Health problems

Even though fruitarianism is often considered to be quite healthy, it can also lead to serious health issues if it is not practiced correctly. Since some nutrients are not available without meat consumption in a sufficient manner, they have to be replaced by using food supplements.

If people miss using those supplements, chances are that those people may suffer from serious nutrient deficiencies, which might eventually translate into serious health issues.

8. May not be suitable for physically exhausting jobs

Opponents of the fruitarian diet also often claim that it might lead to a loss of physical strength. This might be an important downside for people who work in jobs that require plenty of physical work.

Those people urgently need their high levels of energy in order to carry out their job and they might not be able or willing to lose part of their energy due to a switch from a meat-based to a fruitarian diet.

9. Feeling of hunger

Although fruitarians often claim that their diet will be suitable to feel saturated, the opposite is true for many people engaging in this kind of diet. Therefore, many people may feel uncomfortable since they suffer from the feeling of hunger on a constant basis.

You should try it yourself and evaluate if a fruitarian diet will be sufficient in order to feel saturated or not.

10. Social isolation issues

In some areas of our planet, fruitarianism may also not be socially accepted yet. Especially in regions with a high density of meat lovers, you might have a quite hard time to practice your fruitarian diet since people may simply not accept your lifestyle.

Moreover, you might also get socially isolated since many restaurants will not offer food that would be suitable for a fruitarian lifestyle. Thus, depending on your country and your region, you may have problems to integrate into society if you practice fruitarianism.

11. Unnatural diet

Fruitarianism may also be considered kind of unnatural since our ancestors relied on a variety of different foods and our body and our brain evolved millions of years. Thus, refraining from meat and other foods seems to be kind of unnatural and against our natural development.

Is the Fruitarian Diet a Healthy Choice for You?

The fruitarian diet is unique compared to most other diets. While some eating plans may include pre-packaged foods or focus on specific food groups, the fruitarian diet emphasizes just one food group.

The U.S. Department of Agriculture 2020–2025 Dietary Guidelines for Americans recommends consuming a variety of fruits, vegetables, grains, dairy products, and protein each day for a healthy, balanced diet. The key recommendations in the federal guidelines include:

1. A variety of different vegetables including dark, leafy greens, red and orange varieties, legumes (beans and peas), starchy, and others
2. Fruits, especially whole fruits
3. Grains, at least half of which are whole grains
4. Dairy products including milk, yogurt, cheese, and/or fortified soy beverages
5. A variety of protein sources, including seafood, lean meats and poultry, eggs, legumes (beans and peas), and nuts, seeds, and soy products
6. Healthy oils
7. Limited saturated fats, trans fats, added sugars, and sodium

The fruitarian diet does not meet most of these dietary recommendations.3??? While filling half your plate with fruits and veggies, and limiting saturated fats, trans fats, added sugars, and sodium is considered healthy, the fruitarian diet is lacking in vegetables, grains, dairy, protein, and oils.

Whether your goal is to lose, maintain, or gain weight, it's important to know how many calories you should be consuming each day. Most people need around 1,500 calories a day for weight loss, 2,000 calories per day for weight management, and an additional 500 calories a day for weight gain. Of course, this number varies based on age, sex, body type, level of physical activity, and other factors

7-Day Fruit and Vegetable Diet Plan For Weight Loss

After finding out the benefits of the 7-day fruit and vegetable diet, people often consider starting to follow this nutritional plan. But it is not enough to just start eating more vegetables and fruits. To be able to successfully slim down in a healthy way you need a great meal plan for your 7-day fruit and vegetable diet. Here is a well-rounded meal plan you should consider trying out:

DAY ONE

Meal 1: Raspberry Oatmeal

Ingredients:

- ¾ cup oatmeal cooked in 1 ½ cup water
- cup raspberries
- Calories: 310 (per serving)

Meal 2: Whole-Wheat Veggie Wrap

Ingredients:

- 1 8-inch whole-wheat tortilla
- 2 tablespoons hummus
- ¼ avocado, mashed
- 1 cup sliced fresh vegetables of your choice

- 2 tablespoons shredded sharp Cheddar cheese
- Calories: 344.9

Meal 3: Mushroom-Quinoa Veggie Burgers with Special Sauce

Ingredients:

- 1 large portobello mushroom, gills removed, roughly chopped
- 1 cup no-salt-added canned black beans, rinsed
- 2 tablespoons unsalted creamy almond butter
- 3 tablespoons canola mayonnaise, divided
- 1 teaspoon ground pepper
- ¾ teaspoon smoked paprika
- ¾ teaspoon garlic powder, divided
- ½ cup cooked quinoa
- ¼ cup old-fashioned rolled oats
- 1 tablespoon ketchup
- ½ teaspoon salt
- 1 teaspoon Dijon mustard
- 1 tablespoon extra-virgin olive oil

- 4 whole-wheat hamburger buns, toasted
- 2 leaves green-leaf lettuce, halved
- 4 slices tomato
- 4 thin slices red onion

DAY TWO

Meal 1: Huevos Rancheros

Ingredients:

- 2 tsp canola oil
- ½ cup chopped red bell pepper
- ½ cup chopped tomatoes
- 4 cloves garlic, minced
- 1 cup cooked black beans (can be canned, no salt added)
- 1 tablespoon white wine vinegar
- dash of hot sauce
- 2 tablespoons chopped cilantro
- black pepper to taste
- 4 eggs
- 2 tablespoons chopped scallions
- 8 tablespoons salsa
- Calories: 255 (per serving)

Meal 2: Stuffed Potatoes with Salsa & Beans

Ingredients:

- 4 medium russet potatoes
- ½ cup fresh salsa
- 1 ripe avocado, sliced
- 1 (15 ounces) can pinto beans, rinsed, warmed, and lightly mashed
- 4 teaspoons chopped pickled jalapeños
- Calories: 324.4 (per potato)

Meal 3: Beefless Vegan Tacos

Ingredients:

- 1 (16 ounces) package extra-firm tofu, drained, crumbled, and patted dry
- 2 tablespoons reduced-sodium tamari or soy sauce
- 1 teaspoon chili powder
- ½ teaspoon garlic powder
- ½ teaspoon onion powder
- 1 tablespoon extra-virgin olive oil
- 1 ripe avocado
- one tablespoon vegan mayonnaise
- 1 teaspoon lime juice
- 1 pinch of salt
- ½ cup fresh salsa or pico de gallo
- 2 cups shredded iceberg lettuce
- 8 corn or flour tortillas, warmed
- 1-ounce pickled radishes for garnish
- Calories: 360.1 (per 2 tacos)

DAY THREE

Meal 1: Chia Seed Pudding

Ingredients:

- 5 tbsp chia seeds
- 1 1/4 cup almond milk
- ½ tbsp vanilla extract
- Calories: 385 (per serving)

If you tend to let yourself off the hook, raise the white flag when things get tougher than you expected, send yourself on an unconscious binge-eating trip – BetterMe app is here to help you leave all of these sabotaging habits in the past!

Meal 2: Black Bean and Quinoa Salad with Quick Cumin Dressing

Ingredients For the salad:

- 1 cup dry quinoa, rinsed
- dash salt
- 1 cup diced cucumber
- 1 cup diced red bell pepper
- 10-15 basil leaves chopped into a chiffonade
- 1 can black beans, cooked, drained, and rinsed

- 1/4 cup fresh cilantro, chopped

For the vinaigrette:

- 2 tbsp extra virgin olive oil
- 2 tablespoons apple cider vinegar
- 1 tbsp maple syrup or agave
- 2 teaspoons dijon mustard
- 1 tsp ground cumin
- ¼ teaspoon salt
- dash black pepper
- 1 shallot minced (optional)
- Calories: 195.4 (per serving)

Meal 3: Stuffed Pumpkin

Ingredients:

- 1 medium-sized pumpkin or round squash (about 1 kg)
- 4 tbsp olive oil
- 100 g wild rice
- 1 large fennel bulb
- 1 Bramley apple
- 30 g pecans, toasted and roughly chopped
- 1 lemon, zested and juiced
- 1 tbsp fennel seeds

- ½ tsp chili flakes
- 2 garlic cloves, crushed
- 1 large pack parsley, roughly chopped
- 3 tbsp tahini
- Pomegranate seeds, to serve
- Calories: 693 per serving

DAY FOUR

Meal 1: Raspberry Oatmeal

Ingredients:

- ¾ cup oatmeal cooked in 1 ½ cup water
- ? cup raspberries
- Calories: 310 per serving

Meal 2: Stuffed Pumpkin

Ingredients:

- 1 medium-sized pumpkin or round squash about 1 kg
- 4 tbsp olive oil
- 100 g wild rice
- 1 large fennel bulb
- 1 Bramley apple
- 2 garlic cloves, crushed
- 1 lemon, zested and juiced
- 1 tbsp fennel seeds
- ½ tsp chili flakes
- 30 g pecans, toasted and roughly chopped
- 1 large pack parsley, roughly chopped
- 3 tbsp tahini
- pomegranate seeds, to serve
- Calories: 693 (per serving)

Meal 3: Eggplant Rollatini with Cashew Cheese

Ingredients:

- 2 large eggplant, sliced lengthwise into ¼ inch thick slices
- olive oil
- 1 ¼ cups cashews, soaked for at least three hours (or overnight) and drained
- ½ tsp sea salt
- 1 small clove garlic, minced (optional)
- 2 tbsp lemon juice
- ?-½ cup water
- ¼ cup nutritional yeast
- 2 tsp dried basil
- 1 tsp dried oregano
- black pepper to taste
- ½ 10 oz package frozen spinach, defrosted and squeezed thoroughly to remove all excess
- liquid (You may press it firmly through a sieve)
- 1 ½ cups organic, low sodium marinara sauce
- Calories: 187.3 (per serving)

DAY FIVE

Meal 1: Gluten-Free Banana Pancakes, Served with 1 Cup Fresh Berries

Ingredients:

- 1 cup all-purpose, gluten-free flour
- 1 ½ tsp baking powder
- ½ tsp cinnamon dash sea salt
- 1 tsp apple cider vinegar
- 1 ripe banana
- ? cup almond milk
- 1 teaspoon vanilla
- 1 tbsp + 2 tsp melted coconut oil, divided
- a cup of fresh berries
- Calories: 313.75 (per 2 pancakes)

Meal 2: Mango, Kale, and Avocado Salad

Ingredients:

- 1 bunch curly kale, de-stemmed, chopped, washed, and dried (about 6 cups after preparation)
- juice of 1 large lemon

- 2 teaspoons flax or olive oil
- 1 teaspoon sesame oil
- 2 teaspoons maple syrup or agave nectar
- 1 chopped red bell pepper
- 1 cup mango, cut into small cubes
- sea salt to taste
- 1 small Haas avocado, cut into cubes
- Calories: 342.5 (per serving)

Meal 3: Mushroom-Quinoa Veggie Burgers with Special Sauce

Ingredients:

- 1 large portobello mushroom, gills removed, roughly chopped
- 1 cup no-salt-added canned black beans, rinsed
- 2 tablespoons unsalted creamy almond butter
- 3 tablespoons canola mayonnaise, divided
- 1 teaspoon ground pepper
- ¾ teaspoon smoked paprika
- ¾ teaspoon garlic powder, divided
- ½ teaspoon salt

- ½ cup cooked quinoa
- ¼ cup old-fashioned rolled oats
- 1 tablespoon ketchup
- a teaspoon of Dijon mustard
- 4 slices tomato
- 1 tablespoon extra-virgin olive oil
- 4 whole-wheat hamburger buns, toasted
- 2 leaves green-leaf lettuce, halved
- 4 thin slices red onion
- Calories: 394 (per burger)

DAY SIX

Meal 1: Banana and Almond Butter Oats

Ingredients:

- ½ cup old-fashioned rolled oats (such a Quaker®)
- ½ cup vanilla-flavored almond milk
- 1 tablespoon ground cinnamon
- one banana
- 1 tablespoon almond butter
- Calories: 425.1 (per serving)

Meal 2: Kale Salad with Apples, Raisins, and Creamy Curry Dressing

Ingredients For the dressing:

- ½ cup raw cashews or walnuts
- 2 tablespoons lemon juice
- 2 pitted dates
- ½ cup of water
- ½ tsp sea salt
- 2 tsp curry powder

For the salad:

- 1 head kale, de-stemmed, washed, dried, and cut into bite-sized pieces (about 5 cups)
- 2 large carrots, peeled and chopped
- 1 large apple, chopped into small pieces
- ? cup raisins
- ½ cup chickpeas
- Calories: 96.2 (per serving)

Meal 3: Sweet Potato and Black Bean Chili

Ingredients:

- 2 pounds orange-fleshed sweet potatoes, peeled and cut into cubes
- ½ teaspoon ground dried chipotle pepper
- ½ teaspoon salt
- 2 tablespoons olive oil, divided
- 1 onion, diced
- 4 cloves garlic, minced
- 1 red bell pepper, diced
- 1 jalapeno pepper, sliced
- 2 tablespoons ancho chile powder, to taste
- 1 tablespoon ground cumin
- ¼ teaspoon dried oregano
- 1 (28 ounces) can diced tomatoes
- 1 cup water, or more as needed
- a tablespoon of cornmeal
- 1 teaspoon salt, to taste
- 1 teaspoon white sugar
- a teaspoon of unsweetened cocoa powder
- 2 (15 ounces) cans black beans, rinsed and drained
- 1 pinch cayenne pepper, to taste

- ½ cup sour cream, for garnish
- ¼ cup chopped fresh cilantro, for garnish
- Calories: 599.9 (per serving)

DAY SEVEN

Meal 1: Strawberry Oatmeal Breakfast Smoothie

Ingredients:

1 cup of soy milk

- ½ cup rolled oats
- one banana, broken into chunks
- 14 berry (blank)s frozen strawberries
- ½ teaspoon vanilla extract
- 1?½ teaspoon white sugar
- Calories: 236.1 (per serving)

Meal 2: Curry Red Lentil Soup

Ingredients:

- 2 teaspoons olive oil
- 1 head cauliflower, chopped into small florets
- 2 carrots, chopped
- 2 cups boiling water
- 1 cube vegetable bouillon
- 1 (14 ounces) can reduced-fat coconut milk
- a cup of red lentils
- 1 teaspoon garlic powder
- 1 teaspoon dried onion flakes
- a teaspoon of curry powder
- 1 teaspoon paprika
- 1 teaspoon ground turmeric
- ½ teaspoon ground cumin
- 1 bunch kale leaves, stems, and inner ribs discarded leaves coarsely chopped
- Calories: 399.5 (per serving)

Meal 3: Warm Vegetarian Farro Salad with Cauliflower, Pistachios, and Cranberries

Ingredients:

- 2 cups cauliflower florets
- 3 tablespoons olive oil, divided
- 1?½ teaspoons salt, divided
- ¼ teaspoon ground black pepper
- ? cup white wine
- ? cup dried cranberries
- 1 tablespoon honey
- 1?½ cups farro
- 3 cups of water

For the dressing:

- 2 teaspoons lemon juice
- ¼ cup olive oil
- ½ teaspoon salt
- ½ teaspoon garlic powder
- ¼ teaspoon ground black pepper
- 2 tablespoons chopped pistachio nuts
- Calories: 533 (per serving)

1. This refreshing fruit salad is a classic combination that will be the favorite at any potluck or cookout. Serve with a creamy yogurt dressing to take this side (or dessert) to the next level.

Ingredients

- Ingredient Checklist
- 2 cups diced fresh pineapple
- 1 pound strawberries, hulled and sliced
- ½ pint blackberries, halved
- 4 ripe kiwis, peeled, halved and sliced
- 1 cup Lime Yogurt Fruit Salad Dressing (optional; see associated recipe

DirectionsInstructions Checklist

Step 1

Combine pineapple, strawberries, blackberries and kiwi in a large bowl. Serve with yogurt dressing, if desired.

Nutrition Facts

Serving Size: 3/4 Cup Per Serving: 57 calories; protein 1g; carbohydrates 13.9g; dietary fiber 3g; sugars 9.1g; fat 0.4g; vitamin a iu 82.5IU; vitamin c 73.6mg; folate 28.3mcg; calcium 25.8mg; iron 0.5mg; magnesium 18.1mg; potassium 220.6mg; sodium 1.8mg; thiamin 0.1mg. Exchanges:

2. VERY BERRY PALEO VEGAN ICE CREAM

This ice cream recipe is very versitile and yummy! It's Dairy Free, Vegan, Paleo / Primal friend AND is no sugar added.

Ingredients

- cup coconut cream or ½ cup coconut milk
- cup water (or ½ cup water if using coconut milk)
- 100g banana, frozen
- 40g blueberries, frozen
- 20g raspberries, frozen
- 90g strawberries, frozen
- ½ teaspoon vanilla extract

Equipment

- A high speed blender like a Vitamix OR a decent food processor

Instructions

1. Add your coconut cream (or milk) to your blender, add enough water to equal 1 cup of liquid. Add in the rest of your ingredients.

2. Blend on medium speed using plunger if needed (or scrap the sides down if your blender doesn't use a plunger). If using a food processor, pulse several times, scraping down the sides as needed. Blend until creamy and smooth.

3. Serve immediately or you can stick this in the freeze for 30 minutes to firm up more if desired.

Nutrition Information

Serving size: 1 recipe Calories: 300 Fat: 15 Saturated fat: 10 Unsaturated fat: 0 Trans fat: 0 Carbohydrates: 41 Sugar: 23 Sodium: 22 Fiber: 7 Protein: 3 Cholesterol: 0

3. HEALTHY SMOOTHIE RECIPES

These Healthy Smoothie Recipes are all super easy to make and the perfect way to start your day!

INGREDIENTS

- STRAWBERRY BANANA
- 1 banana
- 1 1/2 cups frozen strawberries
- 1 tablespoon chia seeds
- 3/4 cup unsweetened almond milk
- ORANGE GINGER CARROT
- 1 frozen banana, or regluar
- 1 cup fresh orange slices
- 1/3 cup grated carrot
- 1 tablespoon hemp hearts
- 1/2 teaspoon freshly grated ginger
- 1/2 cup almond milk
- 1 handful ice cubes (optional)

MANGO PINEAPPLE

- 1 banana
- 1 cup frozen mango slices
- 1 cup frozen pineapple slices
- 1 tablespoon chia seeds

- 1 cup unsweetened almond milk

KALE AVOCADO CUCUMBER

- 1 banana
- 1/2 cup curly kale
- 1/2 cup peeled cucumber
- 1/4 medium sized avocado
- 1 tablespoon hemp hearts
- 1 handful ice cubes
- LEMON BLUEBERRY
- 1 banana
- 1 1/2 cup frozen blueberries
- 1/4 cup old fashioned oats
- 1/2 teaspoon lemon zest
- 1/2 tablespoon lemon juice
- 1 tablespoons sliced almonds (optional)
- 3/4 cups unsweetened almond milk

CHERRY BEET

- 1 banana
- 1 cup frozen cherries
- 1/2 cup cooked beets
- 1/4 cup old fashioned oats
- 3/4 cup unsweetened almond milk

INSTRUCTIONS

Add all ingredients to a high powered blender and blend until smooth, 30 seconds – 1 minute. Poor into a glass and enjoy.

4. VEGAN FRUIT & NUT BARS

INGREDIENTS

- 6 tablespoons coconut oil (I used JaxCoco)
- 2 tablespoons raw peanut butter
- 4 heaping tablespoons of raw cacao powder
- 2 tablespoons agave (for non vegan use honey or maple syrup)
- pinch of kosher salt
- 1 cup puffed quinoa cereal
- ¼ cup dried cranberries
- ¼ cup chopped pistachio nuts
- ¼ cup shredded unsweetened coconut

INSTRUCTIONS

1. Melt together coconut oil, peanut butter, cacao powder, agave and salt in a microwavable bowl. About 1 minute on high)

2. Stir in the quinoa cereal, cranberries, pistachios and shredded coconut.

3. Pour into a lined loaf pan and chill until set. (about 1 hour)

4. Lift bars from pan, slice and serve.

5. Can be stored in refrigerator for up to one week but they won't last that long so don't even bother reading this instruction.

5. DRAGON FRUIT SMOOTHIE

This vibrant and healthy smoothie works great as a breakfast option or as snack for any time of the day. The deep, rich, pink color comes from the pink dragon fruit

INGREDIENTS

- 1 cup of coconut water
- 1/2 cup orange juice
- 8 oz. crushed pineapples, with the juice

- 1 cup vanilla Greek nonfat yogurt
- 1/4 cup creamy almond butter
- 14 oz. Dragon Fruit
- 1/2 cup blueberries
- 1 tablespoon flaxseed
- 2 tablespoons honey

INSTRUCTIONS

1. Combine all the ingredients in a blender. (Make sure to layer as outlined in the ingredients list so your blender doesn't struggle. Liquids should alway go in first).

2. Blend on medium high or on the smoothie setting on your blender until smooth. If your blender stops, use the tamper provided with the blender to loosen. If you don't have one with your blender, give the mixture a stir with a long metal spoon.

3. Smoothie will store well for up to 3 days. if it separates, shake to combine before serving.

6. APPLE PIE PORRIDGE {RAW, VEGAN, GLUTEN-FREE}

A delicious, warming breakfast that just so happens to be super healthy for you! Suitable for raw, vegan and gluten-free diets.

Ingredients

- 120 ml 1/2 cup almond milk
- 2 tbsp chia seeds
- 2 tbsp almond butter
- 3 dates, roughly chopped
- 1 or 2 tbsp coconut sugar, depending on sweetness desired
- 1/2 tsp mixed spice
- 1/2 tsp ground cinnamon
- 1 green apple, peeled and cored
- Chopped pecans

Instructions

1. Mix all the ingredients, except the chopped nuts, in a blender until thick and smooth.

2. Transfer to a saucepan, stir and heat gently until warm. If you're on a raw food diet, you can

use a thermometer to ensure it doesn't heat above 40c (110f.)

3. Serve with chopped pecan nuts and grate over some fresh apple (I used leftover apple from the core.) Enjoy!

7. 3 INGREDIENT RAW VEGAN CINNAMON ROLLS (LOW-FAT, GLUTEN-FREE)

Ingredients

- 15 organic dates, pitted (I used 3 each of Medjool, Khadrawy, Halawy, Deglet Noor, and Zahidi)*
- 4 large ripe organic bananas
- About 1/2 tsp organic cinnamon + more to top
- Optional: Vanilla, coconut sugar, additional spices.

Instructions

1. Slice the bananas vertically in 3 pieces each.

2. Sprinkle the bananas with cinnamon and place them on a dehydrator at 115F for 6-8 hours.

3. While the bananas dehydrate, create your caramel. Add all of the dates into a high speed blender with a dash of cinnamon, optional vanilla, and 1/4-1/2 cup of water, or as much as is needed to create a thick paste.

4. Once the bananas are able to be handled without breaking, but not completely dry, take slices of and spread the caramel along them. Roll the banana with caramel around itself to form a roll.* Top the rolls with more date caramel if desired. Sprinkle the top with cinnamon.

5. Place back in the dehydrator for 6 hours until warmed through.

Oven

I have not yet tried this recipe in an oven, but this is what I would do if I needed to use one.

Preheat your oven to the lowest heat possible.

Prepare the recipe exactly how it is above, and when placing the bananas into the oven, keep the door cracked open with a wooden spoon for the moisture to be able to escape. Since the heat may be higher, I would do 4-6 hours for the initial dry, then 4-6 for the second. Adjust times as needed.

8. STRAWBERRY BANANA SMOOTHIE

This Strawberry Banana Smoothie is a delicious way to get more fruit into your day. I love having it for breakfast, or as a mid-afternoon snack, because it tastes like such a treat! Even my kids love this one. It's a great "beginner smoothie" if you're trying to make one for the first time.

INGREDIENTS

- 1 cup frozen strawberries
- 1 frozen banana, cut into pieces
- 1 cup milk (I use almond milk)
- 1/2 cup orange juice (or use more milk)
- 1 Medjool date , pitted (or 1 tablespoon honey), if needed for sweetness

INSTRUCTIONS

1. Add the strawberries, banana, milk, orange juice, and date for sweetness, if desired, and blend until smooth. Taste and adjust anything as needed, then serve right away.

2. Leftover smoothie can be poured into mini ice pop molds for a frozen treat later.

9. PUMPKIN SMOOTHIE RECIPE

INGREDIENTS

- 1 cup pure pumpkin puree
- 1 banana (fresh or frozen)
- 3 dates, pitted
- 1 1/2 cups plain almond milk (if allergic to nuts, use any milk you are able to consume)
- 1/2 cup coconut milk
- 1 tsp ground cinnamon
- 1 tsp allspice
- 1/2 tsp ground cloves
- 4-5 ice cubes
- 1/2 tsp raw hemp hearts for garnish

INSTRUCTIONS

1 Combine all ingredients in a blender until smooth.

2 Garnish with hemp hearts

3 Enjoy!

10. 2 INGREDIENT STRAWBERRY BANANA ICE CREAM

2-Ingredient Strawberry Banana Ice Cream-you only need two ingredients to make this healthy ice cream. It is dairy free, vegan, and gluten free. The perfect treat for spring and summer!

Ingredients

- 4 large very ripe bananas
- 1 lb. strawberries washed and hulled

Instructions

1. Peel bananas and slice into ½ inch pieces. Slice the strawberries. Arrange banana slices and strawberry slices in a single layer on a large plate or baking sheet. Freeze for 2 hours or overnight.

2. Place the frozen banana slices and strawberry slices in a food processor or powerful blender. Puree mixture, scraping down the bowl as needed. Puree until the mixture is creamy and

smooth. This will take awhile. Don't worry, the bananas and strawberries will come together. Keep scraping and mixing!

3. Serve immediately for soft-serve ice cream consistency. If you prefer harder ice cream, place in a freezer container and freeze. When ready to serve, let the ice cream sit out for 5 minutes. It will be hard right from the freezer, but it will soften up and you will be able to scoop it.

Conclusion

While the fruitarian diet does provide nutrients from fruits, you likely won't get all the nutrition your body needs. A fruitarian diet lacks protein and healthy fats, as well as vegetables, which are critical to maintaining overall health and optimal bodily function.

Following a fruit-based diet also can also lead to serious cravings for other foods, which may cause bingeing or other forms of disordered eating. Talk to your doctor or a registered dietitian before starting a fruitarian diet. A health professional can help you design an eating plan that will work best for you.

Made in the USA
Coppell, TX
06 March 2022

74575939R10046